ELIXIR OF YOUTH!

Can you devote nine minutes a day to staying young?

If so, these 'Smart Moves' will help you feel better and look better than you have for years. The techniques are non-demanding, easy to follow and they strengthen, stimulate and revitalize your entire body. So forget about repetitious calisthenics, sit-ups, push-ups and expensive exercise equipment — 'Smart Moves' are all you need.

D1150650

Smart Moves

JOHN TIGHE

Foreword by Richard L Saphir, MD

Photographs by Michael Tighe

SPHERE BOOKS LIMITED
30-32 Gray's Inn Road, London WC1X 8JL

First published in Great Britain by
Sphere Books 1983
Copyright © 1981 by John Tighe

SPHERE

Printed and bound in Great Britain by
Collins, Glasgow.

Contents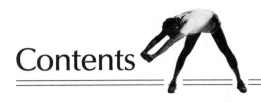

Foreword

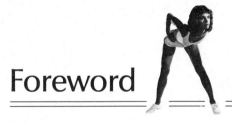

For many years, as a physician and specifically as a pediatrician, I have watched bodies change as minds mature—from the flexible, resilient infant to the more athletic but often stiffer adolescent to the mature adult who is ready to enjoy life to its utmost but cannot because he or she feels "old" and out-of-shape.

Here for the first time are a group of "Smart Moves" that help strengthen, loosen and restore flexibility to your muscles, spine and back. These Smart Moves help you stand straighter and relax more fully by releasing muscular tensions in your neck, shoulders and legs.

These pleasant stretching and twisting movements involve no weights, machines or boring calisthenics. They go far beyond conventional exercise. And they can be used successfully by old and young alike.

I have prescribed them for inflexible adolescents—I have used them myself—and amazingly, they really work!

Staying young is staying flexible. These Smart Moves can truly help you obtain and maintain the flexibility of youth. Use them as part of a daily routine. They can be learned easily and mastered quickly.

I enthusiastically endorse them.

Richard L. Saphir, M.D.

Introduction

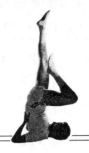

Can you devote nine minutes a day to staying young?

If so, these "Smart Moves" will help you feel better and look better than you have for years.

They're for busy Americans who can't exercise regularly—deskbound executives, white-collar workers who sit in an office all day, mothers who can't get out of the house.

Smart Moves are quite different from conventional exercises. Properly speaking, they're not exercises at all. You can fit them into your spare time at home, or into your coffee break at work. You can do them without working up a sweat. You don't even have to change clothes.

If you enjoy sports—jogging, tennis, skiing—these Smart Moves can help you avoid the stiff joints, sore muscles and pulls that plague weekend athletes. By increasing your flexibility they'll also improve your performance. If you golf, they'll help lower your score by loosening your swing on the first nine.

But primarily they're for people who just don't have time to stay in shape.

They're deceptively simple. Don't let that fool you, though. Just read the instructions and follow them to the letter. If you do, they'll reward you beyond your expectations.

They will make you feel better immediately. They will keep you in shape with a minimum of time and effort. They will help you stay young.

I originally developed these moves for my personal convenience. I was getting old mentally and physically. I was tense, tired, overweight. Like most working Americans approaching middle age, I wanted to stay in shape.

But I wanted to do it in the easiest, quickest way possible.

I began experimenting. I experimented with every fitness program I heard about. I tried running, Judo, Yoga, and Isometrics. I studied everything I could get my hands on.

These Smart Moves are the result, and they speak for themselves.

I'm in better shape now than I was twenty years ago. I'm in better shape than most people half my age.

I'm fourteen pounds lighter and two inches thinner— about the same as I was in college. I not only look good, I feel great.

I'm relaxed. I'm rested. I eat what I like.

I've forgotten what back pain, neck and shoulder tension feel like, even though I spend five days a week at a desk.

A few weeks ago I met my son (he's twenty-five) at a Manhattan restaurant. He introduced me to a friend of his. "This is your father? You're kidding!"

The next day my son's friend stopped by to see him. "Was that really your father? He looks younger than you!"

I loved it! And I love it when friends I haven't seen for a while stop me on the street. "You look different," they say. "You look wonderful. You look younger!"

Looking younger, however, isn't the point. You can do that with makeup and hair coloring.

Physiologically, I *am* younger.

I can plant my palms on the floor without grunting or bending my knees. I can do handstands. I can run miles without breathing hard.

My stomach is flat. Without strenuous exercise or special diet my weight hovers around the ideal prescribed by Dr. George Sheehan, cardiologist and guru of runners. At 56 beats per minute my resting pulse is about the same as an athlete's. *

---

* "Because the athlete's heart is so muscular it can pump the same amount of blood with 50 beats per minute that the average heart pumps with 75 beats. Thus, the athlete's heart will beat 13 million fewer times per year. It works less, rests more, and consequently takes a much

In the past few years I've taught these Smart Moves to a variety of interested people, young and old, individually and in groups, in person and by mail. I've taught them to people in normal health and those with physical handicaps. I've even taught them successfully in classes for the blind.

The techniques are non-demanding and easy to follow. But the underlying principles are so effective that they have been studied at centers for advanced medical research.

They strengthen, stimulate and revitalize your entire body: muscles, glands, nervous system, heart, lungs, arteries. They improve your digestion. They relieve tension, anxiety and depression. They leave you refreshed and relaxed.

So forget about repetitious calisthenics, sit-ups, push-ups. Forget about expensive exercise equipment. Instead of being a chore, these Smart Moves are a pleasure. The results are a pleasure, too.

Last week I had lunch with a business acquaintance I hadn't seen in a couple of years. I was shocked by his appearance. He was fat, flabby, gray. He looked ten years older than me although he's five or six years younger.

But I shouldn't have been surprised. Many people who used to look younger than me, now look older.

In *The Sportsmedicine Book* Dr. Gabe Mirkin calls fitness "The New Fountain of Youth." Based on what these Smart Moves have done for me, I couldn't agree more.

---

longer time to wear out." Gabe Mirkin and Martshall Hoffman, *The Sportsmedicine Book* (Boston, Massachusetts: Little, Brown & Company, 1978), p. 21.

CHAPTER 1

Flexibility, Fitness and Youth

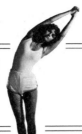

Remember when you were a kid?

You were constantly in motion: running, jumping, skipping, climbing, crawling, doing somersaults. You didn't know the meaning of tension, backache or neck pain. You fell asleep when your head hit the pillow.

Your body was elastic. Your energy was boundless. Within the limits of your strength you could do anything.

Then you grew up. You became sedate. You spent more time sitting than skipping.

You got stiff, put on weight, gradually lost the energy, vitality, potential for vigorous activity—in short the physical *freedom*—you took for granted as a kid.

You assumed this was a "natural" result of getting older. What was happening, however, had less to do with your birthdate than your lifestyle—a sedentary lifestyle you share with 100 million other Americans.

We are nation of sitters—in spite of the fitness explosion. We sit all day at work. We sit going to and from work. We sit all evening in front of the TV set.

We've forgotten that the body is a flexible, versatile mechanism for action and reaction, lifting and leaping, twisting, bending and balancing. Watch a gymnast, a juggler or an acrobat sometime, to appreciate your own potential for flexibility and coordination.

Staying young means staying flexible. You need daily activity to maintain that flexibility. And no matter how brief, it should bring your whole physical mechanism into play—strengthen your muscles, stimulate your glands, organs and nervous system, give your cardiovascular system a workout.

Without this kind of regluar activity you lose muscle tone, your skin sags, your body fat increases, your range of movement decreases. Normal daily activities that should come easily involve effort, sometimes even pain. You get old. Let me demonstrate:

Stand comfortably. Let your head roll backward. Keeping your neck and jaw completely relaxed, roll your head in a 360° circle to the right; then 360° to the left.

Were you able to "let go" and get through the complete cycle without tensing or "clutching"? Did you feel any pain? If so, did you assume this was natural?

Now let your head roll forward on your chest. Relax your neck, shoulders and arms. Keeping your legs straight, let the weight of your head pull you forward and down, and just hang from the waist for a while.

Were you able to hang freely, without pain in your neck, back or legs? Did your knuckles brush the floor?

These simple demonstrations speak more eloquently than I can about what kind of shape you are in.

Mother Nature did not design us for the sedentary life. In the dim past we were prowlers and predators. Our bodies were fine-tuned—constantly poised for attack, defense or flight. Because we ran frequently to pursue game or escape danger, our hearts were strong and healthy. Because we lived one jump ahead of starvation, our percentage of body fat was low. Cholesterol was the last thing we had to worry about.

But the twentieth century does not require us to pursue game or (in general) run for our lives.

Our civilization provides more than we need to eat.

We no longer use our bodies as nature intended.

As Dr. Thomas C. Malone, deputy director of the National Institutes of Health, put it: "The last thing on the agenda of most Americans is to keep this marvelous machine in tune. All the wonderful body machinery we once used to get food and escape predators is no longer utilized."

Does this mean you must run marathons, do chin-ups and push-ups? Not unless you *enjoy* these strenuous activities. In the *Ski Touring Guide* Dr. Thomas J. Bassler says: "Physical fitness does not mean bulging muscles or the ability to lift heavy objects with ease. True fitness is a measure of how well your body functions, of its cardiovascular capability, or how well your heart, lungs and other internal organs act to enable your muscles to perform their tasks."

It means finding a regular system that will keep all your vital body parts functional—your muscles elastic and supple, your spine flexible, your joints lubricated and free, your heart strong, your circulation unobstructed, your digestion efficient.

These techniques are being discovered by growing numbers of Americans. They are used by gymnasts and dancers, by professional football and tennis players, by cardiovascular and stress-reduction clinics, by Yoga and slimming classes, by senior citizens and aspiring actresses—and of course by galloping herds of runners.

In short, they underlie most of today's most effective fitness programs. And they form the basis for this book of Smart Moves.

CHAPTER 2

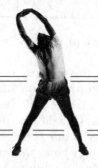

Getting Started

The trouble with many fitness programs is that people start out trying to do too much too fast, get discouraged, and quit. If you've had this experience, the Smart Moves in the following chapter will come as a pleasant surprise.

They're the opposite of the push-pull, grunt-groan exercises Americans are used to. In fact, they're really not exercises but variations of the same cyclical movements, flowing into each other, simultaneously strengthening and relaxing your spine and muscles.

They're ideal for busy people who can't seem to fit even fifteen minutes of exercise into their daily schedules. (Considering that fifteen minutes of conventional exercise requires a special location such as a track or gym; involving total elapsed time of an hour or more to get there and back, get ready, get showered and dressed afterward, it's not surprising that most busy Americans, whether office workers or homemakers, can't find the time.)

Since these Smart Moves can be done wherever you have a few square feet and a few spare minutes, you are more likely to do them. They require no special preparation, equipment or costume. They are carried out in a slow, relaxed manner—the slower and more relaxed, the more effective they become.

Best of all, they make you feel good immediately. Even one set of the two-minute program in the next chapter will give you a lift, restore flagging energy, reduce tension, and make you feel lighter, more resilient, refreshed.

You can do these moves when you first get up in the morning, even after a light breakfast, to provide a reservoir of energy for the day ahead. You can do them after a hard day's sitting, before dinner, or before bedtime to relax your muscles, ease nervous tension and encourage sound sleep.

They're especially good for overcoming the effects of sedentary office work. When you sit for long periods your spine tends to compress. You slump into a curvature that restricts your natural flow of energy. Instead of balancing on top of your spinal column where it belongs, your head slips forward creating a weight imbalance that pulls you forward. To compensate, you unconsciously tighten and shorten the muscles in the back of your neck, creating more tension.

At the same time your legs are not only immobile but bent. Your tight calf muscles and massive hamstrings (the largest muscles in your body) resist the natural lengthening process involved in straightening your legs to stand up.

The *Executive Fitness* newsletter reports that extended sitting causes reduced circulation, weakened muscles, bad posture, backaches, stiffness, fatigue, tension. Furthermore, sedentary workers suffer more illnesses (including heart disease) and are out sick more often than active workers.

The Smart Moves in the next chapter counteract these debilitating effects. They loosen your neck and shoulder muscles, straighten the curvature of your spine, stretch your back and leg muscles, promote deep breathing, exercise your heart and improve your circulation.

They also strengthen your lower back and increase its flexibility. This helps you avoid common back pain and related problems—the category of complaint heard most frequently by doctors in the United States. The more support your back receives, the less strain it endures. The ten Smart Moves in the next chapter not only strengthen the muscles supporting your spine but the spinal column itself.

Each requires a minute or less. You can do all ten in nine minutes. They're divided into two-minute, five-minute and nine-minute programs. If you can't do all ten every day, do the five-minute program. If you can't do the five, do the two-minute program. But . . .

Follow the instructions precisely. Never rush. Always

take your time. The more slowly and *thoughtfully* you carry out these Smart Moves, the more good they will do you.

Don't strain. *Don't* strive for results. Do only what you can accomplish comfortably. Breathe normally, and relax, *relax*, RELAX! This may seem impossible at first, as you learn unfamiliar movements and overcome years of stiffness. But relaxation should always be your goal.

If you do these moves during lunch hour, use them as appetizers—before eating, not after. You'll discover they depress your appetite, and thus help you lose weight.

Your clothes should be loose and non-binding. Practice in shoes, if you like, but make sure neither they nor the surface on which you stand are slippery. Stocking feet, for this reason, can be a problem. You need good traction for the side-to-side twisting movements. I prefer bare feet, the best non-skid "material" I know, particularly on a waxed wooden floor. Admittedly, this may not be practical in an office. But keep it in mind for at home.

And try to get through all ten moves at least once a day, even if you have to split them up.

CHAPTER 3

Ten Smart Moves to Stay Young

The ten Smart Moves in this chapter are designed to be done standing up. This eliminates the need for an exercise mat or similar surface. It also enables you to practice in street clothes if necessary, without worrying about getting dirty from sitting or lying on the floor.

Ideally you should wear comfortable, minimal clothing. Running shorts, T-shirt, and bare feet are my preference. If you are at work, or don't have time to change, regular clothes are fine as long as they don't restrict your movements.

The first three Moves take only two minutes to complete, even though they are carried out quite slowly. If you finish them in less than two minutes, you are doing them wrong.

This two-minute program is for people who have decided they are "just too busy" for anything more ambitious. But hopefully you will find it so rewarding that you will somehow make time for the remaining Moves.

I mentioned earlier that all these Moves are variations of the same slow stretching and twisting motions. So even the two-minute program involves all the muscles of the full nine-minute program.

Move #1 opens up the vertebrae of your lumbar region, frees and strengthens your lower back muscles, eases tension in your neck and shoulders, gently exercises your heart by causing it to beat faster even though you are standing still—as do all these Smart Moves.

Move #2 stretches your massive hamstring muscles, the largest in your body. It loosens tight calf muscles and eases tense neck, back and shoulder muscles. As a tension reliever it is equally effective against early morning stiffness and after a hard day's sitting.

Move #3 relieves tension, stretches and stimulates your arms and shoulders, spine and lower back, calf and hamstring muscles. It promotes overall flexibility, and becomes progressively more effective as you become more flexible.

Since the benefits of these Smart Moves are cumulative, two minutes a day is obviously not going to do you as much good as nine. But it's a start.

If you're too busy to fit even two minutes into your work schedule, do these first three Moves when you get up in the morning. Or after work, before dinner or before going to bed. If time permits, repeat the two-minute program at odd intervals during the day.

On weekends, holidays, vacations, or whenever you have extra time, do all ten Smart Moves in the nine-minute program.

If you have time, make the full nine-minute program part of your daily routine, like meals and brushing your teeth. Practice on an empty stomach. And try to practice at the same time every day, so your workout becomes habitual.

Try never to miss a day. If you must, don't miss more than one day a week. (When you're traveling, for example, there's no excuse to skip a day because you can do these Smart Moves in your hotel room.)

If you are in normal health these Moves should not cause you any problems provided you follow the instructions. And the more carefully you follow them, the more good they will do you.

If you have any doubt about your condition . . . if you have any medical problems such as spinal or back injuries . . . if you have not done any exercise recently, please consult your doctor before undertaking them.

To repeat what I said in the last chapter, relaxation

should always be your goal. Don't push too hard. Don't try to go too fast. Just concentrate on carrying out the Smart Moves slowly and precisely without worrying about results.

You will find that little by little your body will respond by imperceptible degrees, becoming freer, more flexible, more resilient without your noticing it.

SMART MOVE   #1

Throughout this move keep your leg muscles tensed and your hips pushed forward. Otherwise you may lose your balance. Keep your elbows straight out in front of you and arms parallel. Try to keep your neck absolutely relaxed, let your jaw hang slack, and allow your head to roll back freely as you bend backward. If you tried the demonstration in the introduction, you already know that this can be painful at first because of the tension stored up there for years. Do the best you can.

At first, you'll find it difficult to remain in the extreme backward bending position for more than a few seconds. And you'll also notice that your spine begins vibrating. This is no cause for alarm. It's only your spine's natural resistance and the unaccustomed release as it begins opening up.

1. Stand with your feet about a foot apart. Tense your leg muscles. Tighten your buttocks. Push your hips as far forward as possible. Keeping your arms parallel, slowly raise them in front of you, palms down. (See next page.)

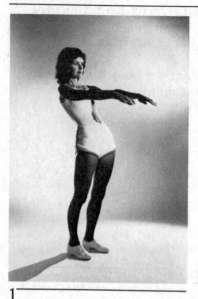

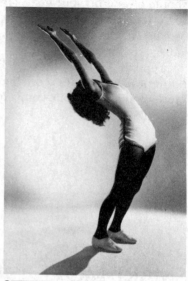

1   2

2. Continue raising your arms overhead. Allow your head to roll back freely. Keep your hips pushed forward and your leg muscles tensed, so as not to lose your balance. Let gravity pull your arms backward and down. Remain this way as long as you can comfortably do so, even though you feel your spine vibrating. Then slowly come up and lower your arms.

SMART MOVE   #2

Sometimes the simplest moves are the most effective. This one consists simply of flopping forward and hanging from the waist, as you did in the demonstration in the introduction. You've probably seen dancers do this a hundred times—in imitation of marionettes, for example.

Their looseness as they dangle between their hips testifies not only to their skill but also their extreme flexibility.

Pay attention to your neck during this move. It is important to keep your neck relaxed throughout. This may be difficult at first because of tension. As you bend forward you may begin to feel a stretching sensation across your back. Resist your natural tendency to ease this discomfort by raising your head and tightening your neck and shoulder muscles. On the other hand, don't bend "actively." Simply allow gravity to pull your torso forward and down, always from the hips. Let the natural resistance of your muscles determine how far down you get. If your initial discomfort is too great, don't fight it. Come right back up.

When you have flopped forward as far as your muscles allow without pushing, mentally check your neck, shoulders and arms for relaxation. They should be limp. So should your hands. Check the small of your back. Try not to let it tighten up. You should feel your hamstrings working as they stretch. You can adjust the degree of hamstring tension by shifting your balance. To ease this tension on your calf muscles and hamstrings, roll your weight back on your heels. To increase it, roll your weight forward. Check your anal sphincter muscle. Make sure it's relaxed. We'll get into a discussion of this muscle and its key role in training you to relax in Chapter 4.

As you roll back up, keep checking your neck, shoulders and arms for relaxation. Let your head roll forward on your chest. Don't bring it up until your body is erect. After you've achieved a degree of flexibility and are able to stay down longer, you'll notice a loosening of your tight spine and lower back muscles while you are flopped forward. You'll feel your spine slowly "giving up," allowing your torso to dip deeper without effort. Eventually your fingertips, then even your knuckles, should rest comfortably on the floor. *Don't push it.* Let the stretch happen by itself.

Smart Move #2, by the way, is used as a preparatory relaxation exercise in acting classes throughout America. You can use it to melt tension too.

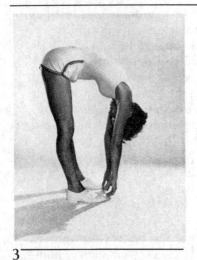
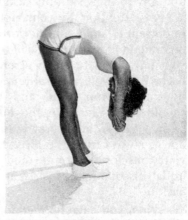

3   4

3. Stand with your feet about a foot apart. Let your head roll forward, and, keeping your legs straight, slowly bend from the hips. Let your arms hang loosely, hands limp. Relax your neck and shoulders. Exhale by contracting your stomach muscles. Inhale by releasing them. Roll your weight forward so that it is on the balls of your feet. Just hang there. Breathe normally. Try to remain for ten breaths or longer. Then slowly roll back up, keeping your neck, shoulders and arms relaxed.

4. As you become more flexible you'll find yourself bending further. Eventually your fingertips will brush the floor. At this stage, simply cross your arms as shown, so you can continue to hang freely.

SMART MOVE #3

This move takes only a minute but relieves tension, stretches and stimulates your arms and shoulders, spine and lower back, calf and hamstring muscles. The more flexible you become, the deeper you get into this move, and the more you get out of it. Carry out each phase slowly, thoughtfully and fully.

You will need good solid traction because the side-to-side twisting will cause your feet to slip if they're not firmly planted. As you twist, keep your feet flat. Don't let them roll outward. Throughout the move, stretch your arms wide but also keep them relaxed.

Sometimes a mental image can help you achieve a physical movement. For this Smart Move, concentrate on your middle fingertips.

Twist from the waist as far to the left as possible. Stay there for a moment, then see if you can go a little farther. Be sure your whole torso is twisting and not just your arms. Your arms should be in a straight line, palms down, parallel to the floor. Don't let your right arm sneak forward as you twist to the left, or your left arm as your twist to the right.

When you bend forward, or sideways toward your knee, the important thing is not how far you bend but how straight your spine remains. This is true of all the remaining moves except #10.

Constantly think of a straight line from your tailbone to your chin. Stretch your chin forward as you bend, and stick your behind out. Keep checking your arms to make sure they are in a straight line, as if there were a bar passing through your shoulders, parallel to the floor. This may seem like a lot of things to keep track of at once, but it will get easier as you become more familiar with the move. Meanwhile, the slower you carry it out the better.

As you bend backward, bend from the hips. Let your jaw remain slack and your head roll back.

On the right and left bends, you should feel a strong pull in the hamstring toward which you are bending. Some strain is all right—it tells you the muscle is stretching. But stop when you encounter pain. Bend as far as you can comfortably, stay there for a while, and come back up. Without noticing, you'll go deeper each day by imperceptible degrees.

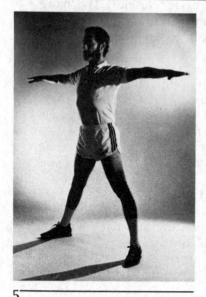
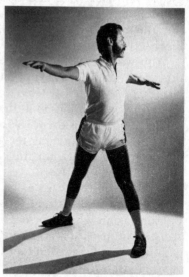

5   6

In the final phase, bending forward, try to sink down between your hips. Don't roll back on your heels. Make sure your weight is far enough forward to produce a good stretch in both legs. And keep your spine straight. Remember to stick out your behind, lead with your chin, and let the bend originate deep in the small of your back. When you've gone as far forward as you can comfortably, try to stay there for a while. Relax your anal sphincter.

5. Stand with your feet planted as wide apart as feels comfortable for you. Keep your legs straight and your knees locked throughout the move. Slowly raise your arms sideways until they form a straight line, fingertip to fingertip, parallel to the floor.

6. Slowly twist your hips to the extreme left. When your hips are fully turned continue twisting your chest to the left, then your shoulders. Look at your left middle fingertip. Pause.

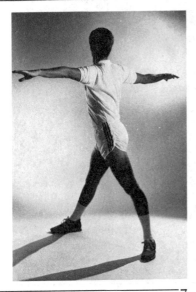

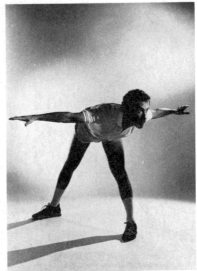

7

8

7. Keeping your torso fully twisted, slowly turn your head and look at your right middle fingertip. Check your arms. Make sure they're straight, fingertip to fingertip. Relax your hands. Keeping your arms parallel to the floor and your eye on your fingertip, slowly rotate your hips, chest and shoulders to the extreme right. Pause.

8. Keeping your torso fully twisted, slowly turn your head back to the left again. Slowly twist to the left and bend toward your left knee. Lead with your chin and stick out your behind. Keep your legs straight, and your arms in a straight line parallel to the floor. Pause.

9. With your hips fully turned to the left and chin extended, slowly straighten up and bend backward, arms still parallel to the floor and palms down. Bend from the hips. Let your head roll backward, jaw slack. Pause. Straighten up and repeat this cycle to the right. (See next page.)

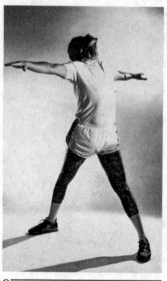

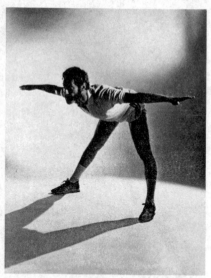

9

10

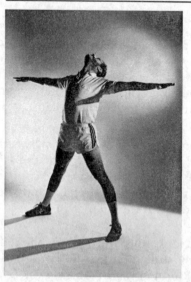

11

10. Straighten up, turn toward the front, and slowly bend forward from the hips. Lead with your chin, keep your back straight, and stick out your behind. Lock your knees and let your weight roll slightly forward onto the balls of your feet. Keep your arms parallel to the floor, palms down. Pause.

11. Slowly straighten up, bend backward, push your hips forward, let your head roll back, and pause. Stretch your arms outward, still parallel to the floor. Straighten up. Lower your arms.

TWO-MINUTE PROGRAM ENDS HERE

SMART MOVE   #4

This move helps reduce tension and tightness in your upper back and shoulders. Keep checking to make sure your palms are solidly placed on your hips (they'll try to come off) and your elbows are pushed backward as far as possible (they'll try to move outward). Resist the tendency to tighten your shoulders and neck as you bend. Keep them relaxed. And don't roll your feet outward. Keep them firmly planted on the floor. As with the previous move, keep your legs straight throughout.

12. Stand with your feet planted comfortably wide apart. Keep your legs straight throughout. Place your hands on your hips and push your elbows back so your bent arms are parallel. Slowly twist to the left and bend from the hips toward your knee. Lead with your chin. Stick out your behind. Keep your legs straight and elbows pushed back. Pause. (See next page.)

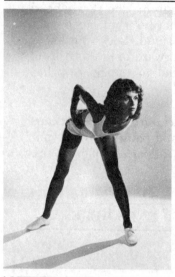

12

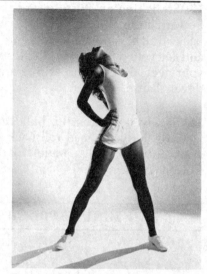

13

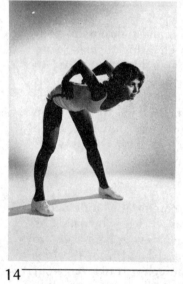

14

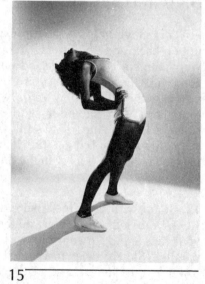

15

13. With your hips fully turned to left and chin extended, slowly straight up and bend backward. Push your hips forward with your hands, push your elbows back, relax your shoulders and let your head roll back. Pause. Straighten up and repeat this cycle to the right.

14. Straighten up, turn front, and slowly bend forward from the hips. Lead with your chin, stick out your behind, push your elbows back, keep your legs straight. Pause.

15. Slowly straighten up, push your hips forward with your hands, let your head roll back, bend backward. Pause. Straighten up and lower your hands.

SMART MOVE   #5

This seemingly simple move is difficult to do properly. But it will reward you by loosening up your lower back and hips as well as strengthening your neck and shoulder muscles. Be sure to keep your feet parallel. Don't let them turn outward. Try to keep your head between your extended arms throughout. At the same time, resist the tendency to bend your arms. Keep them parallel, fully extended, elbows straight. Keep stretching, as though you were pushing with both hands, throughout the move.

16. Stand with your feet parallel, a foot apart. Raise your arms overhead, parallel, elbows straight, palms toward ceiling. (See next page.)

17. Slowly twist to the left and bend from the hips toward your knee. Lead with your chin. Keep your head between

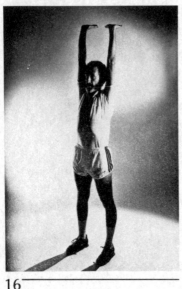
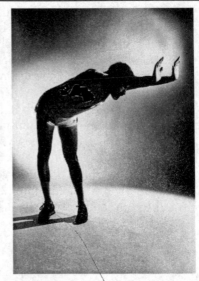

16   17

your arms. Stretch. Push with both hands. Keep your back straight. Stick out your behind. Keep your legs straight. Pause.

18. Keeping your hips fully turned to the left, straighten up and bend backward. Keep your head between your arms. Keep your elbows straight. Push your hips forward. Let your head roll back. Push with your hands. Pause. Straighten up and repeat this cycle to the right.

19. Straighten up, turn front, and slowly bend forward from the hips. Push with both hands. Stick out your behind. Keep your head between your arms, elbows straight and knees locked. Pause.

20. Slowly straighten up. Push your hips forward. Keep your knees locked and your leg muscles tensed. Let your head roll back. Keep your arms parallel, elbows straight. Push with your hands. Pause. Slowly straighten up and lower your arms.

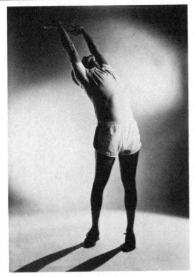

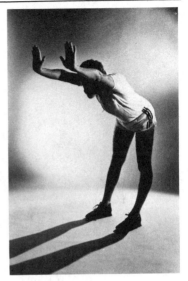

18

19

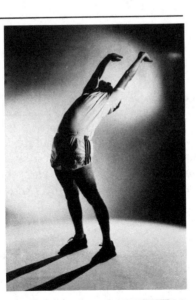

20

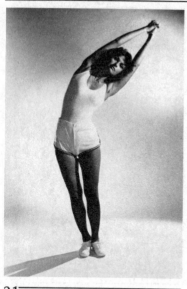
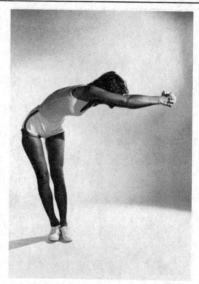

21   22

SMART MOVE #6

This move increases overall spinal flexibility. It's easier than the last one but not as easy as it looks. Concentrate on keeping your arms against your ears, chin out, palms together, back and elbows straight. And don't lose your balance.

21. Stand with your feet together. Raise your arms overhead, interlock your fingers and press your palms together. Keeping your elbows straight and arms against your ears, bend to your left. Pause. Keep your knees together and weight evenly distributed on both feet. Straighten up and bend to your right. Pause.

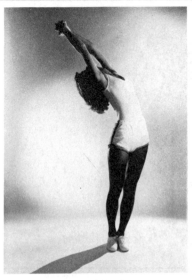
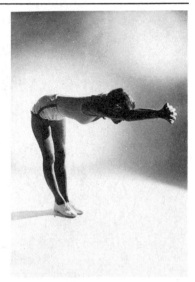

23   24

22. Straighten up, twist your hips to the left, and bend from the hips toward your left knee. Lead with your chin, stick out your behind, keep your legs straight and your arms against your ears. Press your palms together. Keep your elbows straight. Pause.

23. With your hips fully turned to the left, straighten up and bend backward. Keep your arms against your ears and your palms pressed together. Pause. Straighten up and repeat this cycle to the right.

24. Straighten up, turn front, and slowly bend forward from the hips. Lock your knees, stick out your behind, press your arms against your ears, extend your chin. Keep your elbows straight and your chin extended. Pause.

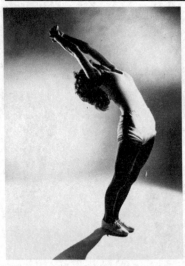

25

25. Slowly straighten up. Push your hips forward, stretch your arms, let your head roll back. Tense your leg muscles. Press your palms. Pause. Straighten up and lower your arms.

FIVE-MINUTE PROGRAM ENDS HERE

SMART MOVE   #7

This move and the two that follow loosen the tight muscles of your upper torso and stretch your leg muscles. The things to concentrate on are keeping your elbows straight, palms pressed together, legs straight and feet firmly planted.

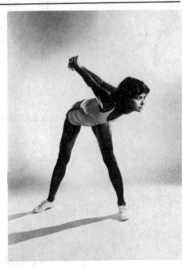

26

26. Stand with your feet comfortably wide apart. Interlock your fingers behind your back. Press your palms together, keep your elbows straight, push your arms away from your back and twist to the left. Bend from the hips toward your left knee. Lead with your chin, stick out your behind, keep your legs straight. Raise your arms as high as possible, keeping your palms pressed together. Pause. Don't roll your weight onto the outside of your feet.

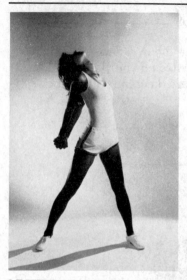

27

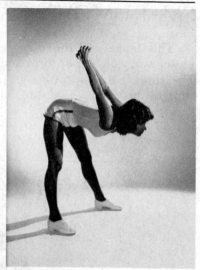

28

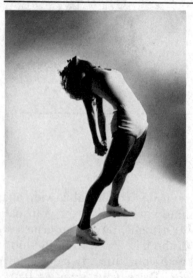

29

27. Keeping your hips fully turned to the left, straighten up and bend backward. Let your head roll back. Push your arms away from your body. Keep your elbows straight and your palms pressed together. Pause. Straighten up and repeat this cycle to the right.

28. Straighten up, turn front, and slowly bend forward from the hips. Keeping your legs straight, lead with your chin, stick out your behind. Raise your arms as high behind you as possible, keeping your elbows straight and palms pressed together. Pause. Don't roll your weight outward on your feet.

29. Straighten up and bend backward. Push your hips forward, keeping your legs straight. Let your head roll back. Push your arms away from your body. Keep your elbows straight and your palms pressed together. Pause. Straighten up and lower your arms.

SMART MOVE #8

If your shoulders and upper torso are too tight to enable you to grasp your elbows at first, grasp your forearms during this move.

30. Stand with your feet comfortably wide apart. Grasp your elbows behind your back. Twist to your left and bend from the hips toward your left knee. Lead with your chin, stick out your behind, keep your legs straight. Pause. (See next page.)

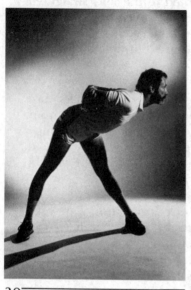

30

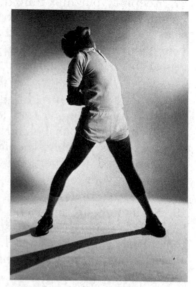

31

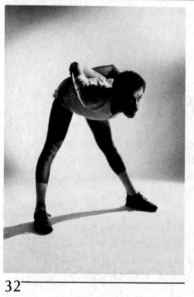

32

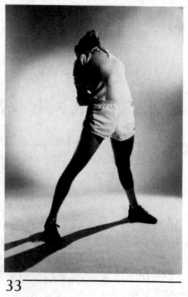

33

31. Keeping your hips fully turned to the left, straighten up and bend backward. Let your head roll back. Pause. Straighten up, and repeat this cycle to the right.

32. Straighten up, turn front, and slowly bend forward from the hips. Keep your legs straight, lead with your chin, stick out your behind. Pause.

33. Straighten up and bend backward. Push your hips forward. Keep your legs straight. Let your head roll back. Pause. Straighten up and lower your arms.

SMART MOVE #9

As with the previous move, if your shoulders are too tight to grasp your elbows, grasp your forearms.

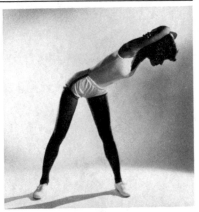

34

34. Stand with your feet comfortably wide apart. Raise your arms overhead and grasp your upper arms just above the elbows, behind your head. Twist to your left and bend

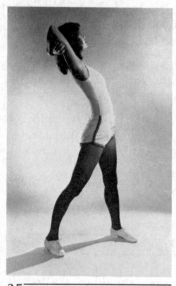
35

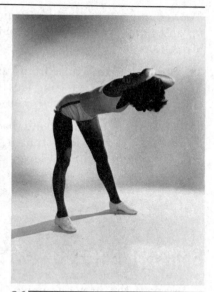
36

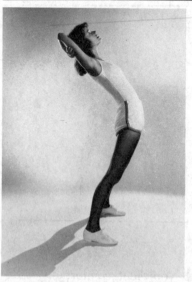
37

forward from the hips toward your left knee. Lead with your chin, stick out your behind, keep your legs straight. Pause.

35. Keeping your hips fully turned to the left, straighten up and bend backward. Push your hips forward. Keep your legs straight. Pause. Straighten up and repeat this cycle to the right.

36. Straighten up, turn front, and slowly bend forward from the hips. Keep your legs straight, lead with your chin, stick out your behind. Pause.

37. Straighten up and bend backward. Push your hips forward. Keep your legs straight. Pause. Straighten up and lower your arms.

SMART MOVE #10

This final move in the series involves continuous movement that brings the whole spine into play, and stretches your leg muscles too. It should be carried out slowly and deliberately, just like the others. Concentrate on stretching and keeping your elbows straight, and be careful not to topple over backward.

38. Stand with your feet comfortably wide apart. Raise your arms overhead, interlock your fingers, turn your palms upward, and push your hips forward. (See next page.)

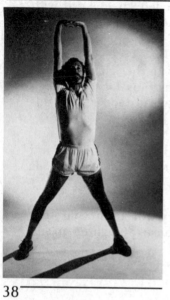

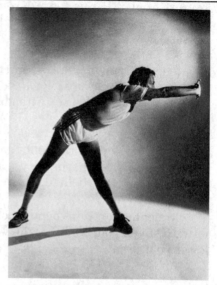

38

39

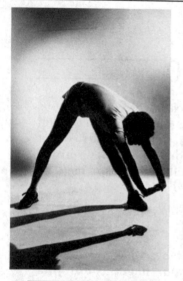

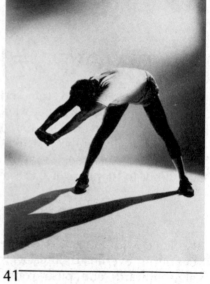

40

41

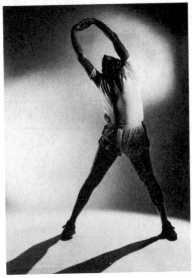

42

39. Twist your waist to the left, stretch and bend toward your left knee. Continue moving down toward your left foot. Keep your elbows straight and your head between your arms.

40. Stretch downward from your hips toward the floor in front of you, palms outward, and continue moving from left to right. Keep your legs straight, stick your behind up, and keep your head between your arms.

41. Continue moving upward in a circular direction, stretching to the right. Keep your legs straight, palms pushed outward, head between your arms and elbows straight.

42. Continue moving upward and back so that you complete a full circle. Push your hips forward, keep your legs straight, let your head roll back. Stretch your arms upward and back, keeping your palms pushing outward and elbows straight. Be careful not to lose your balance. Do two more complete 360° circles. Then do three circles in the opposite direction.

NINE-MINUTE PROGRAM ENDS HERE

CHAPTER 4

Two Smart Moves to Flatten Your Stomach

A. Learning How to Breathe

All the preceding moves help to flatten your stomach. But to a surprising degree the bulge in your midriff is increased by your bad breathing habits.

By improving these habits you can reduce midriff bulge instantly—without dieting or exercise.

Strange as it sounds, most of us don't know how to breathe properly. Instead of filling our lungs, we breathe shallowly. One result is a tendency to slouch, sag and spread.

In *The Human Body* Isaac Asimov writes that during normal shallow breathing we inhale only about 500 cubic centimeters of air. If we inhale voluntarily, we can breathe in 3,000 cubic centimeters—six times the normal amount! Even this, however, is only three-quarters of our lungs' capacity. Another 1,000 cubic centimeters can be breathed in by exhaling completely and by taking the deepest breath possible.

Compare the difference between your breathing when awake and asleep. During waking hours you breathe shallowly, sometimes sporadically. Frequently when you are concentrating on a task, you even hold your breath without realizing it. But during sleep, an involuntary, wiser mechanism takes over. If you share a bedroom you can *hear* the transition from almost inaudible breathing to a deep, steady rhythm as your partner slips into sleep.

By learning to breathe deeply and naturally *all* the time, you'll stand taller, look thinner, feel better.

Feel better? That's an understatement! You'll feel *wonderful*. Deep, natural breathing revitalizes you, relaxes you, relieves nervous and muscular tension—all this in addition to helping you look your best.

The secret is filling your lungs properly with air. When you do, they buoy up your body the way a fishing float buoys up a line and sinker. As your upper torso expands and rises, your mid-section slims and lengthens, your posture improves.

To breathe deeply and naturally, put aside your ideas about inhaling and exhaling. First, exhale by contracting your stomach muscles.

This is contrary to the way most of us think about voluntary breathing. We've been raised on the "take a deep breath" approach: in other words, that *inhalation* is the active part of the breathing cycle, and exhaling the passive part.

Try inhaling now. You'll notice that your natural instinct is to expand your chest. This fills your upper lungs but doesn't utilize the large capacity of your lower lungs. Of course, if you continue to breathe in voluntarily, pushing out your stomach muscles until they are drumtight, you will eventually fill your lower lungs—but with some effort.

Now see how much easier and pleasanter it is to reverse the breathing cycle. Exhale by gently contracting your stomach muscles. This pushes your diaphragm upward, compressing your lower lungs and expelling the air.

To inhale, simply let go. You don't have to do anything. As your abdomen springs back to its released position, your compressed lungs expand creating a vacuum that sucks air deep into your lower lungs.

That's all there is to it. Exhale by gently contracting your stomach muscles. Inhale by letting go.

Get into the habit of breathing this way voluntarily, when you have nothing else occupying your attention. For instance, when you are waiting for a bus or a train, standing in a checkout line, strolling or sitting at your desk.

While you're at it, learn to sit properly. Most of us sit

slumped on our tailbone. To breathe better, improve your posture and reduce your midriff bulge, locate the "sit" bones on the inside of your buttocks. Center your weight squarely over these "sit bones." This alone makes you sit up straighter. Now mentally draw a straight line from the tip of your tailbone, up your spine, along the *back* of your neck to the top of your head (the point where your hair forms a whirlpool). Think of your head as being suspended by a string from that point, like the skeleton in an old-fashioned doctor's office.

Now try to breathe properly. To exhale, gently contract your stomach muscles. To inhale, simply let go.

To intensify your deep breathing, suck in your stomach muscles *hard* as you exhale. Then, as you release them and the air rushes into your lower lungs, continue to inhale, widening and inflating your chest like a balloon.

Try it now. See how good it feels. But stop if you start to get dizzy from the unaccustomed "rush" of oxygen.

Use this intensified deep-breathing exercise to relax before job interviews, at parties where you don't know anyone—whenever you are "uptight." Use it to unwind after a tense day, instead of taking a drink.

To firm and flatten your stomach, use this muscle-contracting move as an isometric exercise. You can do it any place, any time—walking, standing, sitting. Simply contract your stomach muscles as tightly as possible and hold them until you begin to feel strain. Then release. You'll find that you can continue breathing into your upper lungs without difficulty, while your stomach muscles are contracted. You can do this inconspicuous isometric move without anyone being aware of it. Try it several times a day.

Another benefit of voluntary breathing is learning to recognize and release muscular tension—in a way that will surprise you.

The most "neurotic" muscle in your body is your anal sphincter—and the easiest-to-spot sign of tension (once you're aware of it) is a compressed sphincter muscle.

The ringlike sphincter surrounding the anus is usually

the first muscle to "clutch" under stress and the last to relax. This is understandable. Since the anal sphincter's function is to control elimination, we tend to tighten it at the first sign of trouble.

Unless you are unusually relaxed, you are probably tensing your sphincter muscle right now without realizing it. Check and see. Now relax it. Notice the difference.

Once you have acquired this perception you can check for muscular tension and release it at will. Since it's almost impossible to "suck in your gut" without contracting your sphincter—or to let go without relaxing it—voluntary breathing helps train this "neurotic" muscle to relax, and by so doing promotes muscular relaxation in general.

B. A Simple Muscle-Strengthening Move

Strong abdominal muscles act like a girdle in holding your stomach in without conscious effort. This muscle-strengthening move is done lying down. Try to do it at least once in the morning before you get dressed, and again in the evening after work. If you have a private office with a carpet on the floor, try to slip it in during the day, too.

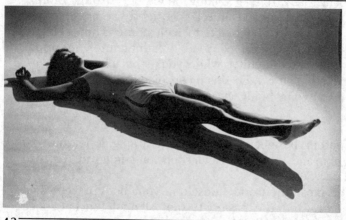

43. Lie on your back, legs together, and let your arms flop comfortably on the floor over your head. Relax. Keeping your legs straight, raise your feet just the slightest bit off the floor—no more than an inch or so. Remain in this position for as long as you can, or until you feel the strain in your stomach muscles. Breathe normally throughout—and try to relax your body completely except for the muscles that are suspending your legs. Check particularly for tension in the back of your neck. When you lower your legs, relax them and let your feet flop out.

CHAPTER 5

More Smart Moves

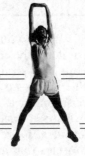

The moves in this chapter extend and deepen the benefits of the preceding moves, and should be carried out in the same unhurried way. In combination with the first ten, they offer an expanded and somewhat more strenuous workout. Since Smart Moves 1 through 10 should be used as a warm-up, I have numbered the following moves 11 through 15, for continuity. These are all done on the floor, so you need some sort of padding such as a carpet or exercise mat. A 2- x 4-foot piece of remnant carpeting with a towel thrown over it is ideal, and can be purchased inexpensively at any carpet store.

SMART MOVE #11

This move is excellent for your lower back. It also relieves tension in your neck and shoulders. Concentrate on keeping your elbows locked throughout.

44. Lie on your stomach, raise your torso and support yourself on your arms. Your legs and feet should be together, arms parallel, elbows straight. Bring your arms back as far as possible toward your body without letting your hips come off the floor. Slowly raise your head and look at the ceiling.

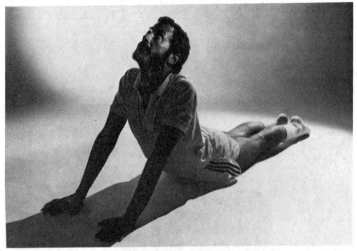

44

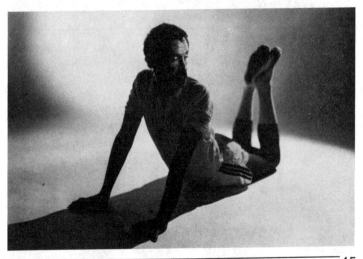

45

45. Keeping your elbows straight, legs together and hips on the floor, bend your knees. Slowly turn your head to the left and try to look at your right heel. Now slowly turn your head to the right and try to look at your left heel. Face front, lower yourself to the floor, and relax.

SMART MOVE #12

This is also very good for increasing flexibility in your lower back.

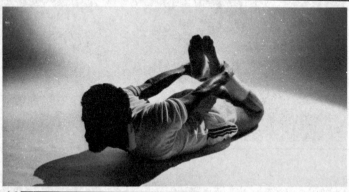

46

46. Lying on your stomach, bend your knees and grasp your ankles. Keep your legs together.

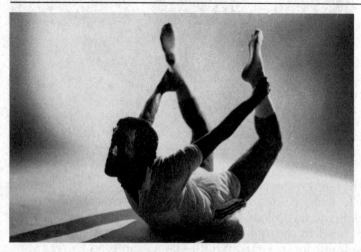

47

47. Slowly raise your head, raise your chest, and look at the ceiling. Now raise your thighs and with your knees together, try to straighten your legs without letting go of your ankles. Widen your legs and continue trying to straighten them. Now relax, slowly come down, and release your grip.

SMART MOVE #13

This move strengthens your spine and back, in addition to promoting overall spinal flexibility. But be careful. You should be able to get up into a shoulder stand without straining. If not, continue doing the previous moves until you can.

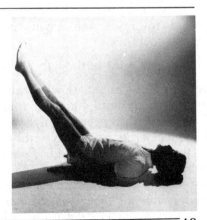

48

48. Lie on your back with your arms by your side, palms down, and legs together. Slowly raise your legs.

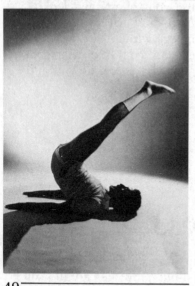

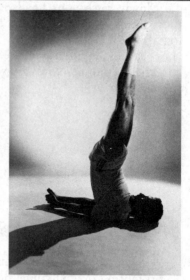

49   50

49. Keeping your legs straight, raise your hips.

50. Align your legs and torso so that they are perpendicular to the floor. Interlock your fingers behind you and press your palms together.

51. Slowly twist your waist to the left.

52. Keeping your legs straight, slowly bring your right leg down across your body until your toes touch the floor to the left of your head. Bring your leg up, twist to the right, lower your left leg across your body until your toes touch the floor to the right of your head. Come back up and straighten your waist.
NOTE: Don't strain to touch the floor with your toes. Stop if you encounter pain and bring your leg back up. Little by little your leg will go further down until your toes touch the floor without effort.

53. Support your hips with your hands so that your legs and torso are again perpendicular to the floor. Bend your left leg forward.

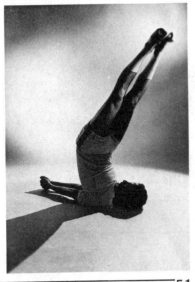

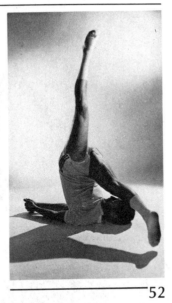

51

52

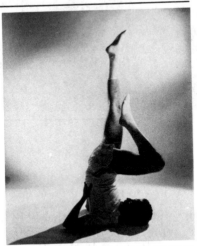

53

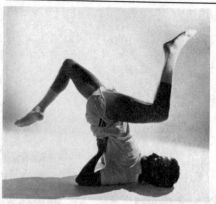

54

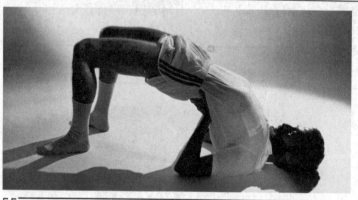

55

54. Supporting your back, let your right leg bend backward until your foot touches the floor.

55. Bring your other leg down so that both feet are planted firmly. Your upper body should be supported by your head, shoulders and arms. Push with your legs and take several deep breaths as outlined in Chapter 4, exhaling by sucking in your stomach muscles and inhaling by releasing them. Then slowly and carefully lower yourself until you are lying full length.

SMART MOVE #14

This move is also effective in loosening and freeing tight back muscles. But approach it with the same caution as the previous one. Don't strain to touch the floor with your toes. Go as far as you can without pain. Eventually your feet will contact the floor without effort.

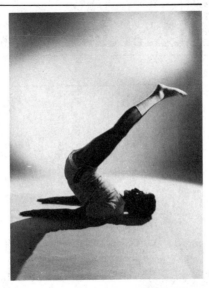

56

56. Lie on your back with your arms by your sides, palms down, legs together. Raise your legs, raise your hips, and bring your legs over your head.

57. Continue until your toes touch the floor. Keep your legs straight and your toes pointed. If you encounter pain in your back before touching the floor, stop at that point, pause, and slowly come down until you are lying full length again. (See next page.)

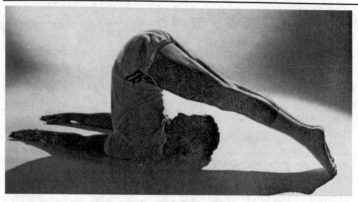

57

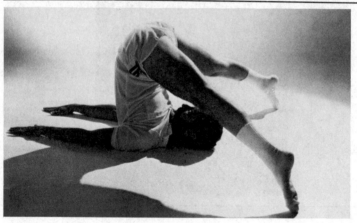

58

58. Widen your legs as far as possible, keeping them straight. Keep your toes on the floor.

59. Bring your legs together and slide them both to the extreme left, then to the extreme right. Keep your legs straight and your toes pointed.

60. Bring your arms overhead and let the toes of each foot rest on your palms. Grasp your toes and pull your legs as wide apart as possible.

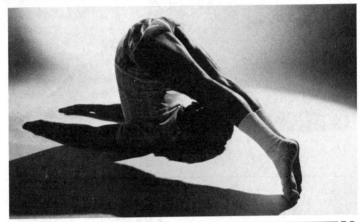

59

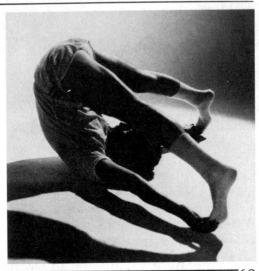

60

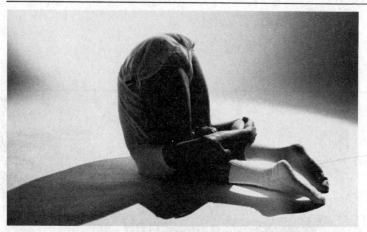

61

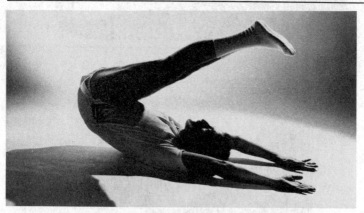

62

61. Bring your knees together, grasp your feet, bend your knees, and pull them in against your shoulders. Wrap your arms around your knees and try to grasp your elbows. Relax and take several deep breaths.

62. Extend your arms overhead. Straighten your legs and roll your torso down until you are lying full length.

SMART MOVE   #15

This move strengthens your back and shoulders, and increases flexibility throughout your pelvic area.

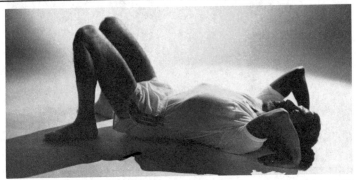

63

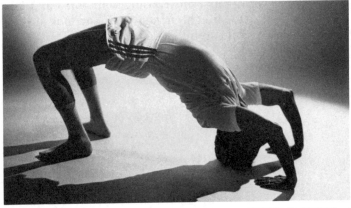

64

63. Lie on your back, bend your knees, and plant your feet comfortably apart and as close to your hips as possible. Plant your palms on either side of your head.

64. Raise your hips off the floor, then your back, and roll onto the top of your head.

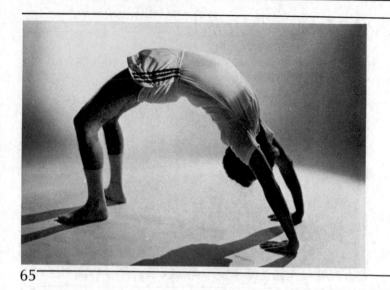

65

65. Push with your arms, raising your torso and head off the floor. Try to straighten your arms and look at the floor. Then slowly and carefully come down.